# Medical Marijuana

Margaret Gramms

Published by Margaret Gramms, 2025.

This book is a personal work based on lived experience

# Table of Contents

◈ Medical Marijuana By Margaret Gramms

What if healing was growing right beneath your feet?

In this powerful and deeply personal book, Margaret Gramms explores the hidden truths, myths, and miracles of medical marijuana — not from a lab bench, but from real life.

From anxiety to chronic pain, from spiritual awakening to the power of feminine resilience, this book unpacks the potential of cannabis as medicine, mystery, and movement. Through vivid stories, grounded insights, and emotional honesty, Medical Marijuana is not just a guide — it's a journey.

# Introduction

Is marijuana, now legalized in many U.S. states, truly a healing remedy — or is it still considered a dangerous drug?

This question remains at the heart of a larger debate about the future of our society, especially the future of our children. As cannabis becomes more accepted and accessible, concerns grow: Is it truly safe? Is it beneficial? And most importantly — what are the long-term effects, particularly on young people?

At what age is it actually safe to use marijuana? Is 18 years old enough? Should it be 21? And even for adults — how does regular cannabis use affect the mind, body, and spirit?

As we legalize cannabis, we must also ask ourselves: What are we truly legalizing — a medicine, or a potential risk?

In this book, we will explore marijuana not only as a substance, but as a symbol — of healing, of power, of controversy, and of cultural transformation. We will examine its uses in folk medicine, its spiritual history, its dangers, and its potential as a natural remedy in a world that is hungry for balance.

# Chapter: How Cannabis Affects the Body — My Intuitive Understanding

I want to begin not with science, but with intuition — with what I feel in my own body and soul.

To me, marijuana is not just a plant. It's a mystery. And I believe it works most powerfully in areas of the body where the muscular system is involved. Why do I say that? I don't know exactly — it's just a feeling. But I truly sense that cannabis affects muscles more than anything else.

It relaxes them. That, I know for sure. Wherever there is tension, cannabis can dissolve it. But what about when muscles are already too loose — could cannabis make things worse? I'm not certain. Maybe it helps, maybe it doesn't.

For example: in gynecological conditions — in the uterus — could marijuana help? Possibly. But what about the heart? I don't believe marijuana is good for the heart muscle. That's just my personal sense. Maybe I'm wrong — I'm open to that. But for now, I have my doubts.

What I do know — without doubt — is that marijuana heals the female orgasm. It softens the body, opens the sensation, deepens the experience. I wouldn't say it "cures" anything — but it brings back feeling, where before there was numbness.

People also say marijuana helps with the brain, or with glaucoma. I don't fully understand how — but I believe it. There is something in cannabis that connects to pressure, to light, to the way the eyes see the world.

# Chapter 2: The Head — Where Everything Begins

The head is the first place we must begin. It is the sacred center of thought, memory, instinct, and choice — the organ given by God to help us navigate life.

As I grow older, I realize more and more that my head has always known the right path. Others may have said different things. I may have misunderstood many messages in life. But the deeper I reflect, the more I see that my own head — my own mind — was guiding me better than anyone else.

Especially now, in this digital age, I finally understand that my mind never betrayed me. It tried to protect me. And the only regret I carry is that I did not listen to it more often.

My way of thinking is unique. My mind never worked like other people's. I often relied on the thoughts and advice of others because I was taught not to trust myself. I was told something was wrong with me. That my brain didn't work like it "should."

But now I see — it was a gift. In the worst moments, when I had no one else, my head saved me. In moments of fear, in moments of danger, I trusted myself — and that saved my life. I only regret every time I asked someone else for advice, when I should have just listened within.

So I choose to begin this book with the head — because that's where life begins. When the mind shuts down, the person disconnects from reality. We call that "madness" or "mental illness," but in truth, it's deeper. A person without mental presence no longer makes choices. They become disconnected from their soul, their purpose.

That's where marijuana enters the story. Can cannabis help the mind?

Can it heal mental pain?

Can it restore a sense of clarity and self-trust?

Let's begin with the head — and see if cannabis is truly a healer... or a deceiver.

# Memory and Mental Clarity: Does Cannabis Numb or Awaken the Mind?

One of the most debated effects of cannabis is its relationship with memory. Does marijuana enhance memory?

Or does it cloud the mind, like a fog rolling in over clear thought?

From my own experience and observation, cannabis seems to create two opposite effects — depending on the person, the dosage, and the moment.

At times, it feels as though cannabis opens a hidden door in the brain. Suddenly, long-forgotten memories resurface. Feelings, scents, and images from the past come alive. Some people describe this as a kind of "emotional memory," where they don't remember exact facts, but they feel what they once felt — more vividly than before.

But at other times, cannabis can soften or block short-term memory. Words slip away. Tasks are forgotten. The mind feels slow, like it's floating in water.

So which is it?

A healer of memory — or a thief of it?

The truth may lie somewhere in between. Cannabis can create a temporary disconnection from logic. It relaxes the brain's filters. This is why people say they feel "creative" — they think outside the usual boxes. But it also means that focused memory tasks, like studying, can become more difficult.

For people with trauma, this disconnection can be healing. Painful memories soften. Emotional pain fades. But for those who need precision and structure, it may feel disorienting.

In essence, cannabis does not destroy the mind — but it changes the channel. It may not turn off the television, but it does switch the program.

For some, this is medicine. For others, it's distraction.

## Emotions, Focus, and the Risks of Disconnection

Cannabis does not act the same for everyone. It touches each person's mind differently — sometimes gently, sometimes like a wave.

Some experience a deep calming effect. Anxiety fades. Worries soften. The inner noise quiets down, like the brain is finally allowed to rest. This is why many people with PTSD, anxiety disorders, or ADHD turn to cannabis — they feel, for once, in control.

But others describe the opposite: racing thoughts, confusion, even paranoia. These reactions are real — and must be respected.

Cannabis can also affect focus and attention. Some people say they become creative, inspired, even visionary. But others lose track of time, forget what they were doing, or struggle to stay present.

One important truth must be spoken:

Cannabis can change your sense of reality.

It may enhance intuition or spiritual vision — but it can also create illusions. Some call them "downloads" from the universe. Others call them hallucinations. Either way, the line between clarity and confusion becomes thinner.

This is why one thing must be very clear:

### It is unsafe to drive a car under the influence of cannabis.

No matter how relaxed or confident you feel — your reaction time slows, your focus may drift, and your sense of space and time can shift.

It is not just illegal in many places — it is dangerous.

Cannabis is a powerful plant. It must be treated with respect, intention, and awareness. It can open the mind.

It can quiet the storm.

But it can also cloud judgment — and even silence the voice of reason if used carelessly.

## Seizures, Panic, and Mental Storms: When the Mind Shakes

For those who suffer from seizures, cannabis can be a gift — but also a risk. Some forms of CBD-rich cannabis have been shown to help reduce seizure frequency, especially in children with rare forms of epilepsy. It works by calming electrical activity in the brain, stabilizing the storm before it rises.

But not all cannabis is the same.

Some strains, especially those high in THC, can actually trigger anxiety, disorientation, or even panic in sensitive individuals. This is especially true for those who are not used to the effects, or who already suffer from mental instability. The difference is in the plant — and the person.

For people prone to panic attacks, small doses of cannabis might bring peace, quiet the mind, and slow down the heart. But large doses, or the wrong strain, can bring on the very panic they were trying to escape.

Cannabis can feel like a warm blanket — or a thunderstorm. I have seen both.

That is why it is so important to understand the individual: their chemistry, their mind, their trauma. One person may find healing. Another may feel terror.

The plant is not good or bad. It is powerful. And power must be used with wisdom.

# Cannabis and Dementia: Searching for Light in the Fog

When someone we love begins to forget, it's more than memory that fades — it's presence, connection, and identity. Watching a parent slip into dementia or Alzheimer's disease is one of the most painful experiences a daughter can face. I know this personally. My own mother has begun to show signs of dementia, and I find myself searching — not just for answers, but for hope.

That is why I turn my attention to cannabis. People ask:

Can marijuana help those with dementia? Can it stop the progression?

Can it bring back something that feels lost? Science does not offer a simple answer.

Some studies show that CBD (a non-psychoactive component of cannabis) may help reduce brain inflammation, which is one of the causes linked to Alzheimer's. There is also evidence that cannabinoids might protect neurons from further damage.

But no one is calling it a cure. Not yet.

What I've seen, and what many caregivers report, is that cannabis can calm agitation. It can help a person with dementia sleep. It can reduce fear and restlessness. Sometimes, just having a few peaceful moments is already a miracle.

It may not restore lost memory, but it can offer comfort. And in dementia care, comfort is sacred.

Still, it must be used carefully. High doses of THC may worsen confusion in some elderly patients. The wrong strain, or too much, might deepen the fog instead of lifting it.

But I hold on to one thought:

If even one moment of peace is possible — if one loving memory can come back, even briefly — that is enough reason to try.

For me, this is no longer a theory. It's a deeply personal journey.

And I believe cannabis, when used with love, respect, and knowledge, may open a small window in a closing world.

# Mental Illness and Cannabis: A Dangerous Door?

Cannabis is often called a medicine — but for some minds, it can be a mirror, a magnifier, or even a trigger.

For people struggling with schizophrenia, bipolar disorder, or borderline personality disorder, marijuana is not always safe. In fact, in certain cases, it can be dangerous.

Let's begin with schizophrenia.

For someone with a vulnerable mind, cannabis — especially high-THC strains — can increase the risk of psychosis. It may create hallucinations, paranoia, or a distorted sense of reality. Even in people without diagnosed schizophrenia, excessive use of cannabis at a young age has been linked to an increased risk of developing psychotic symptoms later in life.

For those who already hear voices, lose touch with reality, or suffer from delusions — cannabis can intensify the chaos. It's not just about getting "high." It's about crossing a line that's already fragile.

With bipolar disorder, the picture is more complex. Some people feel cannabis helps calm their manic energy or soothes their depressive lows. But others find it destabilizes their mood, deepening both highs and lows unpredictably. One moment, they feel euphoria. The next — emptiness.

As for borderline personality disorder, cannabis may offer temporary emotional relief. But it may also increase emotional reactivity, impulsivity, and confusion — the very symptoms that BPD sufferers try to manage.

So what is the truth?

Cannabis is not a cure for mental illness. But it may be a coping tool — for some. And for others — a risk they cannot afford.

It all depends on the person, the dose, and the awareness behind its use.

Mental illness is sacred ground. It deserves more than promises — it deserves honesty.

# Depression, Psychosomatic Pain, and the Silent Suffering

Some pain doesn't show up on X-rays. Some suffering doesn't have a name.
It hides inside the body — but it starts in the mind.
Depression is not just sadness. It is a kind of inner silence, a heaviness that wraps itself around the soul. It slows the body, darkens the thoughts, and makes everything feel far away.
Can cannabis help? Many people say yes.
They describe the first few minutes after a small dose — the way their body softens, their chest opens, and a tiny bit of light returns to the mind. For some, it is the only time they feel joy.
Cannabis doesn't solve problems.
But it can pause the spiral, stop the thoughts that keep repeating, and offer a kind of stillness that antidepressants don't always provide.
But this must be said: cannabis can also become a crutch. Some people begin to rely on it every day to escape reality. Over time, it may make them less motivated, less able to engage with life.
There's a fine line between medication and avoidance.

When it comes to psychosomatic pain — physical pain caused by emotional wounds — cannabis often brings real relief. It relaxes muscle tension, calms the nervous system, and creates a feeling of safety in the body. For trauma survivors, this can feel like a miracle.

But healing must go deeper.

Cannabis can quiet the body — but the soul still needs to be heard. Depression is not laziness.

Psychosomatic pain is not imaginary.

And cannabis is not a cure-all — but it can be a companion on the healing path.

## The Culture of Laziness: When Cannabis Becomes an Excuse

There is a quiet epidemic growing among young people.
It's not just about drugs. It's about disconnect — from responsibility, from purpose, from ambition.
Cannabis, once used as a sacred plant for healing, is now often used as an excuse not to grow.
In many homes, young people gather not to talk, not to connect, but to smoke — again and again — and do nothing.
They call it "chilling," but over time, something begins to rot from the inside.
Motivation fades. Time disappears. Dreams shrink.
This is not medicine. This is avoidance.
I call it the "disease of laziness" — not because these young people are bad, but because they've lost direction. Cannabis becomes a blanket, a cover for pain they can't name, and a tool for comfort that becomes a prison.
Where is the line between help and harm? Here, we must be clear:

Cannabis should not be used to escape life.
It should not be used every day as a substitute for emotion, growth, or courage. This is not healing — it is hiding.
And hiding leads to spiritual starvation.

---

# Autism and Cannabis: A Quiet World, A Different Light

Autism is not an illness. It is a different rhythm of being. A different music that most people don't hear — but it plays constantly in the minds of those who live with it.
Among the many forms of autism, Asperger's syndrome stands out. It is sharp, sensitive, fast-thinking, but often socially invisible. People with Asperger's often feel like aliens — too much, too deep, too "odd" for the world around them.

### "I don't write this as a distant observer. I write it as someone who deeply relates to it, who understands it from the inside out."

There are days when the world is too loud. When the noise of people becomes unbearable.
When a single look, word, or demand can break you.
In such moments, some people on the spectrum turn to cannabis. But does it help?
Some say yes. Cannabis softens sensory overload, reduces social anxiety, and creates a feeling of safety. For women with autism — who often mask their symptoms — cannabis can release the mask, even for a moment, and let them breathe.
For those with Asperger's, it can quiet the spinning mind, ease obsessive thoughts, and open space for rest.
But cannabis also has risks. It can deepen isolation, increase inner spiraling, and disconnect a person from the structure they worked so hard to build.
Because when you're autistic, routine is survival. And cannabis can disrupt that routine.
So again we ask: is it help, or harm?

There is no simple answer.
Cannabis can offer a moment of peace — but it can also pull you further into silence.
For someone with Asperger's, it might feel like relief... or it might feel like disappearance.

## Women, Men, and Cannabis: Two Worlds, Two Reactions

Cannabis touches women and men differently — not only in the body, but in the soul.
For many men, marijuana brings calm, hunger, desire, laughter. It slows them down. It grounds them. It makes them feel present.
But for many women, cannabis does something else entirely. It awakens.
It softens.
It deepens feeling — sometimes to the point of pain. A man may smoke and fall asleep.
A woman may smoke and begin to remember things she forgot — or things she tried to forget. Now add autism to this picture.
Women with autism — especially those who were never diagnosed — often live behind layers of masks. They've been told to smile, to be polite, to act "normal." They carry tension in their shoulders, their voice, their eyes. Even in bed, they may dissociate — not from lack of love, but from too much stimulation.
Cannabis, for them, can be a key.
It can unlock the body. It can bring back sensation, pleasure, even orgasm — in someone who thought she was broken.
But sometimes, it unlocks too much.
The trauma comes. The emotions rush in. She might cry, shake, collapse into silence — and the man beside her doesn't understand why.
Because to him, cannabis is pleasure.

To her, it is revelation. This is the gap.
A woman may want to talk after. A man may want to sleep.
A woman may relive her past.
A man may just enjoy the moment. This difference is not about fault.
It's about nervous systems, trauma, and depth.
Especially in autistic women — who already live in a world that feels too much, cannabis can either be a balm or a storm.

**A Message for the Future: Let Us Not Hide, Let Us Guide** Cannabis is now legal in many places — and I believe that is the right direction. Why?

Because when something is illegal, it doesn't disappear. People still use it — they just use it in the dark, with shame, with secrets, with fear. And that, I believe, is more dangerous than the substance itself.

Let us be honest: most drugs, unlike alcohol, were originally created for healing. They were not meant to destroy — they were meant to relieve pain. Even marijuana, long feared and criminalized, holds medicinal properties. We should not ignore that.

But we must also be wise.

Just because something is allowed does not mean it should be abused. Just because something is natural does not mean it is harmless.

For example: you can smell alcohol on someone. A drunk person behind the wheel is easier to catch.
But cannabis? No smell.
And yet, it too slows the mind, the reflexes, the connection to the road.
So no — I do not believe anyone should drive under the influence of cannabis.

But I also believe that for someone suffering from anxiety, trauma, or emotional pain, cannabis might be the bridge that helps them return to life. The answer depends not just on the plant — but on the person.

What I want more than anything is to protect our children. They are our future. They are the soul of what comes next.

But hiding the truth from them will not protect them.

Lying will not protect them.

Only honesty — and example — can. Let them see us think.

Let them hear us question.

Let them feel safe to ask, to learn, and to choose.

Because when we forbid everything without explanation, we don't just ban — we break trust. We build fear. And fear can lead to rebellion, to trauma, to silence.

We are not our parents.

We are trying to raise a new generation with less shame, less fear, more choice. I have seen too many young people fall into depression.

Not because of cannabis — but because of loneliness, confusion, and the emotional inheritance of generations who never talked about anything.

Now we must talk.

We must guide our children, not punish them. We must give them tools, not threats.

We must offer them truth — and trust them to decide. That is what this book is for.

Not to glorify. Not to condemn.

But to understand.

# Chapter 3: Oxygen: The Breath of Life, and the Risk of Cannabis

When someone dies in a hospital bed, it is often not because of pain — but because they can't breathe.
Their oxygen drops. Their lungs are too tired. And their body lets go.
In nursing homes, we see it every day.
Low oxygen — low energy — and the beginning of the end. So what does cannabis do to oxygen levels?

## ➤ First, the hard truth:

Smoked cannabis reduces oxygen intake.
It irritates the lungs, slows the exchange of gases, and can temporarily lower oxygen saturation, especially in older or already weak patients.
For people with COPD, emphysema, asthma, or heart failure — this can be dangerous. This is why cannabis should never be smoked by people with oxygen dependency.
Even vapor may be risky in fragile lungs.

## ➤ But now, the nuance:

Some forms of cannabis — especially CBD oil — may help the body use oxygen more efficiently, by relaxing the nervous system and reducing the oxygen demand caused by panic or breathlessness.

For example:

- A patient struggling to breathe may panic
- Panic increases heart rate → more oxygen needed
- CBD may calm the system → less oxygen demand

So cannabis doesn't increase oxygen, but it may help the body require less. That is the difference.

In palliative care, where oxygen levels are already low, some caregivers use cannabis oil to help a patient feel calm, breathe slower, and die in peace — not in fear.

## The Breath and the Smoke: Cannabis and the Lungs

When we speak, sing, cry, or even breathe — we use the most sacred passage in the body: the throat and the lungs. This is where life enters. This is where voice is born.

But what happens when smoke enters that space? Can cannabis heal the very organs it passes through?

Let us begin with truth.

## ➤ Dry Cough and Mild Throat Irritation

Cannabis — especially when smoked — can actually cause dry cough or throat irritation in sensitive people. For this reason, it is not recommended for treating basic laryngitis or pharyngitis. In fact, in raw smoke form, it may make these conditions worse.

However, if used in vaporized or oil form, cannabis may help in another way — by relaxing the muscles in the throat and calming overactive coughing. It won't cure infection, but it can reduce spasms and make breathing more comfortable.

Acute bronchitis caused by infection should not be treated with smoked cannabis. But again, in non-smoke form, CBD-rich cannabis may help by easing inflammation in the bronchial tubes and making the coughing less painful. Still, it's not a cure. It may offer symptomatic relief, not healing.

### ➤ Asthma

It may sound strange, but some people with asthma report that low-dose cannabis vapors help them breathe more easily. This is likely due to the plant's bronchodilator effect — it can open airways slightly. However, for asthmatics, smoke is dangerous. So this must only be considered with extreme care, and never in raw inhalation form.

## ➤ Emphysema

In emphysema, where lung tissue is permanently damaged, cannabis does not reverse the damage. However, some people find that edible forms of cannabis help with shortness of breath and reduce anxiety that comes with gasping or struggling to breathe.

## ➤ Tuberculosis

Cannabis is not a treatment for TB. It does not fight the bacteria. However, in advanced stages, it may help relieve pain, calm fear, and ease breathlessness. But it must not replace real medical care.

## ➤ Lung Cancer

This is where things get complex. Some studies suggest that cannabinoids (especially CBD and CBG) may have anti-tumor properties. In animal studies and some lab tests, cannabis compounds slowed the growth of certain cancer cells — including in the lungs.

But there is no approved cannabis cure for lung cancer. Still, for pain, nausea, sleep, and appetite during treatment, cannabis can offer true relief. It may not heal — but it may help someone keep going.

---

### ◈ Summary of Benefits

- Helps with: chronic cough (non-infectious), bronchial spasm, asthma (vapor form only), anxiety during emphysema, symptom relief in lung cancer

• Does not help: direct healing of infections (like pharyngitis, TB), tissue regeneration in emphysema, bacterial diseases

# Chapter 4: Digestive Tract(esophagus-rectum).

Where cannabis can help — and where it can backfire. (◈ = possible benefit / ◈ = risk or limitation)

- ◈ Δ$^9$-THC relaxes the lower esophageal sphincter, making acid reflux and esophagitis more likely.
- ◈ Smoking or vaping dries the mouth, fuels bacterial plaque, and worsens chronic halitosis.
- ◈ Cannabinoid-hyperemesis syndrome (recurrent, violent vomiting after long-term heavy use) further injures the esophagus.

No proven upside for the esophagus or bad-breath control.

## Stomach (gastritis, ulcers, cancer)

- ⯑ Balanced THC/CBD formulas ease chemotherapy-triggered nausea and vomiting, including in gastric-cancer patients.

- ⯑ In animal and early human studies, $CB_1$ activation cuts acid output and shields the gastric lining; low-dose CBD has sped healing of small ulcers.

- ⯑ Population data link heavy cannabis use to higher hospitalization rates for peptic-ulcer disease.

- ◈ THC slows gastric emptying and, with chronic overuse, can trigger hyperemesis.

---

- ◈ Acute and recurrent "cannabis-induced" pancreatitis is being reported with growing frequency; no robust evidence for anti-inflammatory benefit.

## Small Intestine & IBD (Crohn's, ulcerative colitis)

- ◈ Clinical trials show pain, cramping, diarrhea, and overall quality-of-life scores improve with THC or whole-plant inhalation. ◈ Endoscopic healing, however, usually does not follow.
- ◈ Symptom relief may mask a silent flare and delay medical care.

- ◈ Pre-clinical work points to CBD, CBG, and mixed phytocannabinoids inducing apoptosis and slowing growth of colorectal-cancer cells; early human data are still exploratory.

- ◈ A 2025 epidemiologic study found heavy users with established colon cancer had dramatically worse five-year survival (likely tied to immunity, adherence, or comorbidities).

- ◈ For diagnosed patients, cannabis can blunt pain, nausea, and cachexia during chemo or radiation.

- ◈ Dronabinol and other agonists slow gastric emptying, inhibit colonic tone, and may worsen gastroparesis or chronic constipation when overused.

- ◈ In carefully titrated doses, the same motility dampening can calm spasms and nausea in functional dyspepsia or refractory gastroparesis.

## Bottom line

Cannabis in digestive disease is, at best, adjunctive: it can ease pain, spasm, nausea, and treatment side effects, but it does not replace proton-pump inhibitors, biologics, surgery, or oncologic protocols. Any trial run should be physician-supervised, with close watch for reflux, delayed emptying, hyperemesis, or pancreatitis.

# Chapter5: Cardiovascular System

The Heart, the Pressure, and the Pulse

The heart is the engine of life. It carries our blood, our breath, and often, our emotions. A strong heart keeps everything moving. A tired one — can bring everything to a stop.

Cannabis affects the heart — but not always in the ways people expect.

In this chapter, we will explore how cannabis interacts with the cardiovascular system. Where it may help, where it may harm, and what we still do not know.

The Heart, the Pressure, and the Pulse

The heart is the engine of the body. It keeps the blood moving, supports every organ.

In this chapter, we will explore the possible benefits, the risks, and what we still do not know when it comes to marijuana and heart health.

---

## ⯑ Possible Benefits (⯑):

1. High Blood Pressure (Hypertension):

Some studies suggest that CBD (non-psychoactive component of cannabis) may reduce stress and anxiety, which can lead to temporary lowering of blood pressure. However, this effect is mild and not a replacement for proper medical treatment.

1. Stress-related Chest Tightness:

CBD may help ease tension in the body, which can reduce non-cardiac chest pain caused by anxiety or nervous system overactivity.

1. Post-Heart Attack Anxiety or Insomnia:

In very low doses, cannabis may help some people relax and sleep after experiencing a heart attack, especially if anxiety is high. This should only be used under strict medical supervision.

---

## ◈ Serious Risks (◈):

1. Fast Heart Rate (Tachycardia) and Arrhythmia:

THC — the psychoactive part of cannabis — can increase heart rate, cause palpitations, and trigger irregular heartbeats in sensitive individuals. This can be dangerous, especially for those with pre-existing heart conditions.

2. Heart Attack Risk:

In elderly or at-risk individuals, cannabis use (especially smoking) has been linked to a higher risk of heart attack, particularly in the first hour after use. This is due to increased heart rate and oxygen demand.

3. Blood Pressure Drops (Hypotension):

Cannabis can sometimes cause a sudden drop in blood pressure, leading to dizziness, fainting, or falls — particularly in older adults or those already on medication.

---

## Summary

Cannabis and the heart do not always go well together.

- If used with caution, certain CBD forms may offer mild support with stress and anxiety.

- However, for people with serious heart conditions, cannabis (especially high-THC) can be dangerous.
- Smoking, in particular, carries serious cardiovascular risks.

This is not a system to experiment with.
The heart deserves respect — and decisions made with full understanding.

# Chapter 6: Urinary System

The Kidneys, the Bladder, and the Body's Natural Filters

The urinary system is the body's internal filtration system. The kidneys remove toxins from the blood. The bladder stores and releases waste. When this system suffers, the whole body feels it — through pain, swelling, infection, or toxic overload. What role can cannabis play here?

Let's explore what it may support — and where it has no proven benefit.

Absolutely — here is the section in clear, professional English, fully focused on the urinary system:

# Urinary System

The Kidneys, the Bladder, and the Body's Natural Filters

The urinary system serves as the body's essential filtration pathway. The kidneys cleanse the blood, balance fluids, and regulate electrolytes. The bladder stores waste until it is released. When these organs are stressed or failing, the entire system can suffer — from discomfort and inflammation to dangerous toxicity.

Can cannabis support urinary health? Let's look at what is known.

## ◈ Possible Benefits (◈):

Chronic Kidney Disease (CKD):
Cannabis does not cure kidney disease. However, it may help with symptom management, including:

- Chronic pain
- Nausea
- Insomnia
- Loss of appetite

CBD, in particular, has anti-inflammatory properties that may ease overall discomfort. Some patients on dialysis use cannabis to feel more relaxed or to reduce pain during and after treatment.
Bladder Pain Syndrome (Interstitial Cystitis):
In some cases, cannabis may reduce nerve sensitivity and inflammation in the bladder region, leading to less pain and urgency.
Urinary Tract Infections (UTIs):
Cannabis does not fight infection. It does not replace antibiotics. However, it may reduce bladder cramping, discomfort, and muscle tension during recovery.
Dialysis:
Cannabis may offer emotional and physical relief during dialysis. It may ease:

- Muscle cramps

- Stress
- Fatigue
- Anxiety

But it must be used carefully, as kidney patients often have complex medication regimens.

## ◈ Known Risks (◈):

- Kidney strain from high-THC cannabis: In rare cases, excessive THC use may stress kidney function, especially if combined with dehydration or other drugs.
- Unpredictable interactions with dialysis medications.
- Smoking cannabis is not recommended for kidney patients due to its impact on oxygen and cardiovascular strain.

## Summary:

- Cannabis may offer relief for pain, anxiety, sleep, and discomfort related to urinary diseases or dialysis.
- It does not treat infections or restore kidney function.
- Always use non-smoke forms (oils, tinctures, capsules) and only under medical supervision for kidney patients.

# Chapter 7 : Reproductive System

Masculine and Feminine Responses to Cannabis

# Male Sexual Health: Strength, Sensation, and Uncertainty

## MEDICAL MARIJUANA

When it comes to male sexuality, cannabis has a mixed reputation. Some men say it enhances sensation, increases pleasure, and helps them relax into intimacy. Others report the opposite — that cannabis causes low libido, delayed ejaculation, or erectile dysfunction.
So what is the truth?

- In small amounts, cannabis may relieve performance anxiety and increase sensitivity.
- In larger or chronic use, it may reduce testosterone levels and decrease sperm count.
- Long-term heavy use has been linked to lower sexual drive and motivation in some men.

For men struggling with premature ejaculation, cannabis may delay climax, which can be helpful. But for others, it may reduce intensity or emotional connection.
So for male sexuality, cannabis can be a pleasure — or a block. It depends on the man, the dose, and the intention.

---

## Female Sexual Health: Awakening the Body, Reclaiming the Self

For women, the effects of cannabis on sexuality are often more emotional, energetic, and sensual. Especially in women with high sensitivity, anxiety, trauma history, or autism, cannabis may help unlock the body in a gentle and profound way.
Women report:

- Increased sensation and body awareness
- More intense and prolonged orgasms
- Easier emotional surrender during intimacy
- A feeling of being present inside the body, not disconnected

Cannabis seems to soften resistance — physical, emotional, and even subconscious.
For women who have never orgasmed, or who struggle to feel safe during sex, cannabis may act as a bridge — helping the body relax, open, and receive.

However:

- Too much THC may cause emotional flooding, paranoia, or disconnection.
- In some women, cannabis may increase sensitivity to the point of discomfort.

So again — dose matters, intention matters, and listening to the body matters.

---

## ⟐ Summary

- ⟐ For men: may reduce anxiety and delay climax
- ⟐ For men: may decrease testosterone and desire in high doses
- ⟐ For women: may enhance orgasm, body awareness, and emotional openness
- ⟐ For women: risk of emotional overload or discomfort in high doses

Cannabis is not just about sex.
It's about feeling — fully, deeply, safely. And for some, that begins in the bedroom.

Softness, Surrender, and Coming Back to the Body

For many women, the greatest barrier to pleasure is not the body — it's the mind.

Anxiety, trauma, pressure, shame, fear of judgment, dissociation... all of these live inside the female body like locked doors. And even when the desire is there — the body might not follow.

Cannabis, in the right moment and amount, can become a key.

Women across cultures have reported that cannabis:

- Increases genital sensitivity
- Enhances full-body awareness
- Deepens emotional presence
- Softens internal resistance
- Helps reach or intensify orgasm
- Allows surrender without fear

Especially in women who have experienced sexual trauma, chronic pelvic tension, or sensory processing disorders (including autism), cannabis can gently reconnect the mind and body — something years of therapy alone might not accomplish.

This is not about addiction or dependence. This is about awakening.

Many women have never felt a "true orgasm." Some have never been able to surrender to it. Cannabis may lower the internal noise long enough for her to finally feel safe — and fully alive in her own body.

But caution is important:

- Too much THC can lead to emotional overwhelm
- Not every strain enhances sexuality — some dull it
- Each body is different — trial, patience, and intention matter

The female orgasm is not a performance. It is not linear.
It is not for anyone else's validation. It is a return to self.

Cannabis is not a shortcut — but for some women, it is the door that was never open before.

# Female Hormones & Reproductive Balance

Cycles, Transitions, and the Feminine Endocrine Flow
The female body is governed by intricate hormonal rhythms — a dance of estrogen, progesterone, and other messengers that shape mood, fertility, sexuality, and overall well-being.
Cannabis may offer subtle support at various stages of this journey.

## ⯑ Possible Benefits (⯑):

1. PMS and Menstrual Cramps:

THC and CBD may help relieve:

- Uterine cramps
- Irritability and anxiety
- Breast tenderness
- Headaches during menstruation

Some women use CBD oils or cannabis suppositories for pain and pelvic relaxation.

2. Hormonal Mood Swings:

Fluctuating hormones (especially before menstruation or during perimenopause) can cause mood instability. Cannabis may support:

- Calmness
- Emotional regulation
- Reduced anxiety

3. Menopause Symptoms:

Cannabis, particularly CBD-rich blends, may help with:

- Hot flashes
- Night sweats
- Sleep problems
- Mood swings and anxiety

4. Fertility Stress:

While cannabis is not recommended during active attempts to conceive, it may help reduce stress and cortisol, which can negatively affect fertility in high-stress women. (Use with caution; see below.)

---

## ⟐ Risks and Limitations (⟐):

- High-THC use may disrupt ovulation if used daily or in high doses
- Regular cannabis use may reduce fertility in both women and men
- Not recommended during pregnancy or breastfeeding
- Can affect hormone-sensitive conditions like PCOS or endometriosis differently for each woman

## Summary:

Cannabis may offer gentle support during hormonal transitions, especially for:

- Menstrual pain

- Menopause-related sleep or anxiety
- Emotional regulation

But it should be used with mindfulness, especially if fertility or hormonal disorders are a concern.

# Chapter 8: Endocrine/Thyroid System

Metabolism, Energy, and the Balance Within

The thyroid is a small gland with a powerful role. It regulates metabolism, controls energy levels, affects mood, weight, temperature, and hormonal balance throughout the body.

When the thyroid is out of balance, everything feels off — from chronic fatigue and depression to anxiety, insomnia, weight gain, and brain fog.

Can cannabis help?

Let's explore what is currently known about cannabis and thyroid health.

## ◈ Possible Benefits (◈):

1. Anxiety and Insomnia from Hyperthyroidism:

In cases of overactive thyroid, many people suffer from restlessness, rapid heart rate, and difficulty sleeping. Low-dose cannabis, especially CBD, may help calm the nervous system and improve sleep quality.

2. Chronic Pain and Mood Support in Hypothyroidism:

In underactive thyroid (hypothyroidism), patients often report joint pain, sluggishness, and depressed mood. Cannabis may help improve energy, reduce inflammation, and elevate mood
— though it does not treat the root cause.

3. Autoimmune Thyroiditis (Hashimoto's):

Some early research suggests that CBD may have an effect on the immune system's inflammatory responses, potentially easing autoimmune flare-ups. However, there is no clinical proof that cannabis slows the disease process.

## ◈ Known Risks (◈):

- Cannabis may interfere with thyroid medication absorption, especially if smoked.
- THC may increase anxiety in sensitive individuals with thyroid imbalances.
- No studies confirm that cannabis directly affects thyroid hormone levels (T3, T4, TSH).

## Summary:

- Cannabis does not treat thyroid disease directly, but may help relieve related symptoms like anxiety, pain, fatigue, and sleep disturbance.
- It is not a replacement for thyroid hormone therapy.
- Always consult a doctor when combining cannabis with thyroid medication.

# Endocrine System

Hormones, Sugar, and Inner Balance

The endocrine system controls the body's internal messages: metabolism, energy, reproduction, sleep, and stress — all through the language of hormones. When this system falls out of balance, everything feels misaligned.

Diabetes is one of the most common and serious endocrine disorders, affecting the body's ability to regulate blood sugar.

Can cannabis help?

Let's explore what science and experience suggest.

## ◈ Possible Benefits (◈):

1. Blood Sugar Regulation (Type 2 Diabetes):

Some studies show that cannabis users may have lower fasting insulin levels and improved insulin sensitivity. This is likely due to anti-inflammatory properties of cannabinoids like CBD, which may help reduce insulin resistance in Type 2 diabetes.

2. Nerve Pain (Diabetic Neuropathy):

Cannabis, especially topical or oral CBD and THC blends, may help reduce:

- Nerve pain
- Tingling and numbness in feet or hands
- Sleep disruption caused by pain

3. Inflammation and Weight Balance:

Chronic low-grade inflammation plays a role in diabetes and obesity. Cannabis may support inflammation control, helping restore metabolic balance in some people.

4. Appetite and Mood:

For diabetic patients with appetite loss or depression, cannabis may offer mild appetite stimulation and mood support, especially during medication side effects or dietary challenges.

## ◈ Risks and Limitations (◈):

- Increased appetite ("the munchies") from high-THC cannabis can lead to overeating and poor food choices, which may worsen blood sugar control.
- Cannabis can interact with diabetes medications, affecting metabolism and blood pressure.
- Long-term effects on pancreatic function are not yet fully understood.

- Smoking cannabis may reduce cardiovascular health — already a concern for diabetics.

---

## Summary:

- Cannabis does not cure diabetes, but it may support symptom relief and metabolic regulation in Type 2 cases
- It may help manage nerve pain, inflammation, and sleep disturbances
- Caution is required to avoid negative dietary effects or medication conflicts

Always consult with a healthcare provider before combining cannabis with insulin or other hormonal medications.

# Graves' Disease & Hyperthyroidism

Autoimmunity and the Overactive Thyroid

Graves' disease is an autoimmune condition where the immune system mistakenly stimulates the thyroid gland, causing it to enlarge and overproduce hormones. This leads to a state of hyperthyroidism — too much energy, anxiety, insomnia, fast heartbeat, and weight loss.

In rare cases, this overactivity can also affect the thymus gland (located in the chest), particularly in children and adolescents. The thymus may grow abnormally in response to immune signals.

## ◈ Does cannabis help?

Current research is limited, but CBD (a non-psychoactive compound in cannabis) may help in two ways:

## ⟐ Possible Benefits (⟐):

- Reduces autoimmune inflammation that may contribute to thyroid overactivity
- Helps calm the nervous system, reducing anxiety, heart palpitations, and insomnia

- May support hormonal balance indirectly by affecting stress hormones (like cortisol)

## ◈ Risks and Limitations (◈):

- Cannabis does not treat the root cause of Graves' disease
- It may interfere with thyroid medications like methimazole or beta-blockers
- High doses of THC may worsen heart symptoms like tachycardia

## Summary:

- Cannabis, especially CBD-rich formulas, may help manage symptoms of hyperthyroidism (anxiety, sleep, stress)
- But it is not a cure for Graves' disease and must be used cautiously
- Always consult a doctor before mixing cannabis with thyroid medication

## Myasthenia Gravis & Multiple Sclerosis

**The human body can mistakenly attack itself. In conditions like Myasthenia Gravis (MG) and Multiple Sclerosis (MS), the immune system interferes with how nerves and muscles communicate.**

- **Myasthenia Gravis causes muscle weakness, especially after activity**
- **Multiple Sclerosis causes nerve damage, leading to fatigue, vision loss, numbness, and coordination issues**

## ◈ Can cannabis help?

Research is still developing, but many patients report relief with certain cannabis compounds.

## ◈ Potential Benefits (◈):

- Muscle relaxation and spasm relief (especially in MS)
- Reduced inflammation in the nervous system
- Better sleep and reduced anxiety
- Improved appetite and less fatigue

CBD and balanced THC:CBD formulas are most commonly used.

## ◈ Risks and Concerns (◈):

- Cannabis does not stop disease progression
- May interact with immune-suppressing medications
- High THC may cause dizziness or worsen fatigue in some cases

## Summary:

Cannabis may offer symptomatic relief for some patients with:

- Muscle stiffness
- Fatigue
- Pain
- Anxiety

But it should be part of a carefully supervised treatment plan, especially in complex autoimmune diseases like MG and MS.

- Spasticity Relief: Cannabis can reduce muscle stiffness and involuntary spasms, a common symptom in MS.

- Neuropathic Pain Reduction: Many MS patients experience nerve pain, which cannabinoids (especially THC and CBD) may relieve.

- Bladder Control and Sleep: Some report better control over bladder function and improved sleep quality.

- Fatigue and Mood: May help reduce fatigue and support mental health by decreasing anxiety and depression.

---

## Lupus (Systemic Lupus Erythematosus)

- Anti-inflammatory Effects: Lupus involves widespread inflammation. CBD, in particular, has anti-inflammatory properties that may help calm the immune response.

- Pain Management: Cannabis can assist in reducing joint pain, muscle aches, and chronic fatigue.

- Sleep Support: Many lupus patients struggle with insomnia, and cannabis may help promote deeper sleep.

- Autoimmune Modulation: Some research suggests cannabinoids may regulate immune system overactivity, though more studies are needed.

- Appetite Stimulation: THC is well-known for increasing appetite ("the munchies"), which is crucial for patients suffering from HIV-related weight loss or wasting syndrome.

- Nausea and Vomiting Relief: Cannabis can help manage nausea caused by antiretroviral medications.

- Neuropathy Relief: Many HIV patients suffer from peripheral nerve pain, which cannabis may relieve without the risks of opioids.

- Mental Health Support: Cannabis may also help reduce anxiety, depression, and feelings of isolation in long-term HIV survivors.

Medical Marijuana for Muscular Disorders
Medical marijuana has shown potential in managing symptoms of various muscular diseases, including conditions such as multiple sclerosis (MS), muscular dystrophy, amyotrophic lateral sclerosis (ALS), and spasticity-related disorders. Here's how it may help:

- Muscle Spasms and Spasticity Relief:

One of the most well-documented benefits of medical cannabis is its ability to reduce muscle stiffness and spasms, especially in MS patients. THC and CBD may help relax overly contracted muscles and reduce involuntary movements.

- Pain Reduction:

Many muscular disorders are accompanied by chronic pain. Cannabinoids can alter pain perception in the brain and reduce inflammation in muscles and nerves, offering a natural pain relief option without opioids.

- Improved Sleep and Mobility:

Muscle pain and spasticity often interfere with sleep and daily movement. Cannabis may promote deeper sleep and improve mobility by reducing discomfort.

- Neuroprotective Properties:

Some studies suggest cannabinoids may protect nerves from further degeneration in progressive conditions like ALS or MS, though more research is needed.

- Mood and Mental Health Support:

Chronic muscular illnesses can lead to depression or anxiety. CBD and low-dose THC may help stabilize mood, reduce anxiety, and support emotional well-being.

# Chapter 10: Ophthalmic System

Vision, Pressure, and the Inner Eye

The eyes are more than sight — they are gateways to the soul, windows of perception, and mirrors of internal pressure.

## ◈ Cannabis and Glaucoma

Cannabis is widely known for its ability to reduce intraocular pressure, making it a potential support in treating glaucoma. Studies confirm that THC can lower eye pressure for several hours — but the effect is short-lived and requires frequent dosing, which can lead to unwanted side effects.

◈ Helpful short-term, but not a long-term solution

◈ Not a substitute for prescribed glaucoma medication

## ◈ Other Eye Conditions

There is no strong evidence that cannabis helps with:

- Cataracts
- Macular degeneration
- Eye infections or burns

However, cannabis may help with eye strain, tension headaches, or visual stress related to screen use and fatigue.

# Chapter:11 Skin and Hair

The Surface of Emotion, Immunity, and Identity

The skin is the body's outer voice — it shows what we feel, fight, and carry. The scalp and hair reflect vitality and internal balance.

## ◈ Possible Benefits (◈):

1. Eczema and Psoriasis:

Topical CBD creams may help reduce inflammation, redness, and itchiness by calming the immune response in chronic skin conditions.

2. Acne and Inflammation:

CBD has antibacterial and anti-inflammatory properties that may reduce breakouts when applied to the skin.

3. Hair Loss (Alopecia):

Though not proven to regrow hair, cannabis oils may help reduce stress-related shedding and improve scalp circulation.

4. Wound Healing:

Some balms infused with cannabis are used for burns, minor cuts, and skin irritation, offering pain relief and faster healing.

---

## ⟐ Limitations:

- Cannabis does not cure infections or fungal diseases.
- THC products may worsen oily skin or cause sensitivity in some individuals.
- Effects on hair growth are not clinically confirmed.

The Surface of Emotion, Immunity, and Memory
The skin holds more than our shape — it holds our stories. It reacts to stress, emotion, trauma, and imbalance. Hair, too, reflects the inner world: stress, hormones, nutrition, and vitality.
Cannabis may offer support in certain skin and scalp conditions — but not all. Below are the conditions where cannabis is most relevant.

# ⯑ Effective Applications (⯑)

1. Eczema (Atopic Dermatitis):

CBD-enriched creams and salves have shown promise in reducing itchiness, redness, and inflammation, especially in stress-aggravated cases. The calming properties help soothe overactive immune responses.

2. Psoriasis:

As an autoimmune skin condition, psoriasis involves inflammation and overproduction of skin cells. CBD and other cannabinoids may reduce flare-ups, calm the immune response, and ease skin discomfort.

3. Wound Care & Burns:

Cannabis-infused ointments and balms are sometimes used in minor burns, skin abrasions, and small cuts. They may help with:

- Pain relief
- Anti-inflammatory response
- Faster surface healing

4. Hair Loss (Stress-Induced Alopecia):

While cannabis doesn't directly regrow hair, it may support:

- Reduced hair shedding caused by stress and anxiety
- Improved blood flow to the scalp via oils and massage
- Emotional calming, which affects hormone-sensitive hair loss

## ◈ Limitations and Risks (◈)

- Cannabis does not treat bacterial or fungal skin infections
- High-THC topicals may irritate sensitive skin or worsen oiliness
- No confirmed evidence that cannabis stimulates new hair growth

This system — like many others — benefits most from topical, low-dose, and non-psychoactive cannabis applications.
It is not about getting high.
It is about restoring peace to the body's outer boundary.

## ⟐ What About Nails?

Cannabis doesn't directly affect nail growth the way it might influence skin or hair — but it may still have indirect benefits through its overall effect on health and inflammation.

## ◈ Possible Benefits (◈):

- Reduced inflammation: If nail issues are linked to autoimmune conditions (like psoriasis or lupus), CBD may help reduce flare-ups and tenderness around the nails.
- Stress relief: Chronic stress can worsen nail-biting, cuticle damage, or poor nail health. Cannabis may help by calming the nervous system, which indirectly supports self-care and healing.
- Improved sleep and nutrition: Good sleep and nutrient absorption are essential for nail strength. If cannabis helps with sleep or digestion, it might also benefit nail health over time.

## ◈ Limitations (◈):

- Cannabis does not strengthen nails directly
- It has no proven effect on nail growth rate
- It won't reverse fungal infections or trauma to the nail bed

## Bottom Line:

Cannabis is not a nail-strengthener — but if the problem is rooted in stress, autoimmunity, or poor sleep, it might offer gentle support through whole-body balance.

# Chapter 12: Forms and Types of Medical Marijuana

Consumption Methods and Cannabis Varieties

Medical marijuana is not only smoked. Today, cannabis can be used in many different forms depending on a person's needs, preferences, and health condition.

## Forms of Consumption:

1. Smoking (joints, pipes, bongs)

○ Fast effect, but not ideal for lung health.

2. Vaping (pens, cartridges)

○ Cleaner than smoking, works quickly, but still involves inhalation.

3. Edibles (cakes, candies, oils, drinks)

○ Delayed effect (30–90 minutes), but lasts longer. Often used for sleep, pain, or anxiety.

4. Tinctures and oils (under the tongue)

○ Moderate onset, good for precise dosing.

5. Capsules and tablets

○ Convenient and discreet, used as regular medication.

6. Topicals (creams, balms)

○ For local pain, muscle soreness, or skin inflammation. No "high."

## Types of Cannabis:

There are two main natural types:

- Sativa
  - Uplifting, energizing, focus-enhancing
  - May cause anxiety or overstimulation in some people

## ⚖ Choosing the Right Type

Some strains are hybrids, combining effects of both sativa and indica. The right choice depends on:

- The condition being treated
- Time of day (energizing vs. calming)
- Individual sensitivity to THC or CBD

Always start low and go slow, especially with edibles.

## ◈ Final Note

Medical marijuana is not just a medicine — it is a tool. It can help, but only if used with knowledge and responsibility. Not everything that's natural is harmless, and not everything that's controlled is dangerous. It's all about understanding and balance.

# Last chapter: Accessing Medical Marijuana in California

How the System Works for Real People
In California, medical marijuana has been legal since 1996 under Proposition 215. The process is simple — but for many people, it still feels overwhelming. Some don't know where to start.
Others feel too shy, isolated, or afraid to talk about it. Here's a simple guide to how it works:

## ◈ Step-by-Step: How to Get a Medical Marijuana Recommendation

1. Find a licensed physician

You don't need your regular doctor. Many licensed cannabis doctors are available online or in clinics.

1. Get evaluated

The doctor will ask questions about your condition (pain, anxiety, insomnia, etc.). You don't need to "prove" your illness with documents — just explain honestly.

1. Receive your recommendation

If approved, you'll get an official letter or card. This allows you to buy from licensed medical dispensaries.

1. Use safely and legally

Medical patients can buy higher-strength products and carry more cannabis than recreational users.

---

## ⟐ For People Who Feel Alone

You are not alone. Many people suffer in silence — especially with conditions like chronic pain, PTSD, or depression. It's okay to ask for help. You don't need to tell your family. You don't need to post about it. This is about your health, your healing, your right.

## ⚖ Final Note

California law protects medical privacy. Your employer, landlord, or school will not be notified. You have the right to choose your path to wellness — quietly, privately, and legally.

www.ingramcontent.com/pod-product-compliance
Lightning Source LLC
LaVergne TN
LVHW060041210926
848481LV00013B/3924